PCOS COOKBOOK SOLUTION

James E. Godinez

Disclaimer

This book contains information for general informative purposes only; it's not intended to be taken as professional advice. Since the author is not a lawyer, he or she cannot offer specific legal advice or vouch for the truthfulness, completeness, or applicability of the data presented.

Table of content

Introduction

Embarking on the journey of living with PCOS is like navigating through a stormy sea. The waves of emotions can be overwhelming, with each crest and trough representing the highs of hope and the lows of frustration. This book, "PCOS Cookbook Solution," is your lighthouse in the tempest, guiding you towards a haven of understanding and control.

In the introduction, we lay the foundation for a transformative experience. It's a heartfelt welcome to readers who may feel isolated by their condition, offering them a sense of community and understanding. We acknowledge the silent struggles, the unspoken fears, and the shared dreams of wellness that unite us all.

We begin by exploring the emotional rollercoaster that is PCOS. It's a candid conversation about the condition, not just as a physical ailment but as an emotional one that affects every aspect of life. From the anxiety of symptoms to the hope of recovery, we delve into the stories that make each journey unique.

The power of food is then introduced as a central theme. It's not just about the nutrients and the calories; it's about the moments of joy when savoring a meal that's both delicious and healing. It's about the empowerment that comes from knowing you're nurturing your body with what it truly needs.

This introduction is an invitation to turn the page on PCOS, to start writing a new chapter in your life where you're in control. It's a promise that through the pages of this book, you'll find more than recipes—you'll find a path to a healthier, more vibrant you.

It's a message of hope: You are not alone on this journey. Together, we'll discover how to live a healthy life with PCOS, one meal at a time. Let's embrace this journey with open hearts and a spirit of resilience. Welcome to "PCOS Cookbook Solution"—where your healing begins with every bite.

Chapter 1: The PCOS Pantry - Your Foundation for Healing

Imagine a pantry that's more than just shelves stocked with food. It's a sanctuary, a place where each item is a building block for your health and well-being. This is the vision of Chapter 1: "The PCOS Pantry," a cornerstone of your journey towards healing from PCOS.

In this chapter, we delve into the heart of your kitchen, where the battle against PCOS begins. It's an intimate space where choices are made that can either fuel the disorder or foster recovery. We understand that these choices are not just practical but deeply emotional. The foods you stock in your pantry are not mere commodities; they are symbols of hope and agents of change.

"The PCOS Pantry" is about creating a nurturing environment that supports your body's needs. It's about replacing the confusion and chaos with clarity and purpose. We'll guide you through selecting ingredients that are powerful allies in your fight against PCOS, ingredients that are known for their anti-inflammatory properties and hormone-balancing effects.

As we walk you through the essentials of a PCOS-friendly pantry, we share stories of women who have stood where you stand now. Their struggles, their successes, and their insights become a part of your narrative, offering comfort and motivation. You'll learn that each spice jar, every grain of whole rice, and even the bottle of olive oil you place on your shelf carries with it a promise—a promise of a healthier tomorrow.

This chapter is not just about lists and recommendations; it's a heartfelt dialogue about transforming your relationship with food. It's about embracing the power you have to influence your health positively. With every item you add to your pantry, you're taking a step towards empowerment, towards a life where PCOS does not define you.

By the end of this chapter, your pantry will be transformed into a treasure trove of healing, each item handpicked by you, for you. It's a testament to your commitment to yourself, a tangible reflection of your journey to wellness. Let "The

PCOS Pantry" be the first chapter of your success story, where every ingredient is a beacon of hope, and every meal is a step closer to the life you deserve.

Stocking Up for Success - The First Step to Empowerment

As you stand in the aisle of the grocery store, surrounded by an abundance of choices, the act of stocking up your pantry becomes more than just a routine—it becomes the first step towards reclaiming your health and writing a new story for yourself. "Stocking Up for Success" is the subchapter where we begin this transformative journey together.

This subchapter is an intimate exploration of the emotional process behind selecting the foods that will fill your shelves and, more importantly, nourish your body in its fight against PCOS. It's about making choices that resonate with your goals, your dreams, and the life you envision for yourself beyond PCOS.

We understand that each item you place in your cart carries with it the weight of your hopes. The olive oil glimmers with the promise of heart health, the bags of quinoa whisper of balanced blood sugar levels, and the fresh vegetables are vibrant with the potential for hormonal harmony. These are not just ingredients; they are symbols of your dedication to a healthier you.

"Stocking Up for Success" is a heartfelt narrative that acknowledges the courage it takes to start this journey. It's about the quiet moments of victory when you choose almond milk over dairy, recognizing the small decisions that lead to big changes. It's about the sense of pride that comes from filling your space with foods that empower you, foods that are your allies in the battle against PCOS.

In this subchapter, we share stories of triumph and encouragement. You'll read about others who have stood where you stand now, who have felt the uncertainty you feel, and who have emerged victorious. Their experiences become a source of strength and inspiration, a reminder that you are not alone in this.

As you turn the pages, you'll find yourself immersed in an emotional and practical guide to building a pantry that supports your journey. It's a guide that's been crafted with care, understanding, and a deep respect for the path you're on.

By the end of "Stocking Up for Success," you'll have more than just a well-stocked pantry—you'll have a treasure chest of hope, a testament to your commitment, and a clear vision of the success that lies ahead. Let this be the first of many steps towards a life of wellness, balance, and joy.

The Anti-Inflammatory Staples - Nourishing Your Body and Soul

In the quiet sanctuary of your kitchen, there lies a powerful arsenal against PCOS: the anti-inflammatory staples. These are not just ingredients; they are the guardians of your well-being, the silent warriors that combat inflammation and bring balance to your body. "The Anti-Inflammatory Staples" is a subchapter that speaks to the heart of healing, offering solace and strength through nutrition.

This subchapter is a tender narrative that intertwines the science of anti-inflammatory foods with the emotional journey of living with PCOS. It's about the hope that stirs within you when you discover the healing potential of turmeric, the comfort you find in the rich omega-3s of flaxseeds, and the peace that comes with sipping on green tea.

We delve into the stories behind these staples, each one a testament to nature's power to heal. You'll learn about the ancient roots of ginger, revered for its medicinal properties, and the humble blueberry, bursting with antioxidants.

These staples are your companions on a path to wellness, each one chosen for its ability to soothe, heal, and restore.

"The Anti-Inflammatory Staples" is an emotional guide that acknowledges the struggles you face with PCOS. It's about the frustration of managing symptoms and the yearning for relief. But it's also about the triumphs—the joy of finding natural remedies that work for you and the empowerment that comes from taking control of your health.

As you read through this subchapter, you'll feel a connection to the foods you eat. You'll understand that each spice, each seed, and each leafy green is more than just a part of your diet; it's a part of your life's tapestry, woven with threads of hope and resilience.

By the end of this subchapter, you'll have a pantry filled with more than just food; you'll have a collection of stories, a repository of healing, and a newfound sense of agency. Let "The Anti-Inflammatory Staples" be a source of comfort and a beacon of hope, guiding you to a life where PCOS is no longer a defining factor, but a condition you live with in harmony and health.

Balancing Hormones with Every Bite - A Symphony of Healing

In the delicate dance of hormones that orchestrates the rhythm of your body, every bite you take is a note in the symphony of healing. "Balancing Hormones with Every Bite" is a subchapter that resonates with the profound and personal journey of restoring harmony within your body.

This subchapter is a heartfelt exploration of how the foods we choose can be powerful conductors in the symphony of our endocrine system. It's about the emotional connection we forge with our meals, the comfort we find in the familiar flavors, and the hope we place in each nutrient-packed ingredient to bring balance to our hormones.

We delve into the emotional stories of those who have walked the path of PCOS, sharing their struggles with hormonal imbalances and their triumphs in finding equilibrium through mindful eating. It's a narrative that celebrates the small victories, like the joy of a balanced meal that leaves you feeling satisfied and at peace, without the highs and lows of blood sugar spikes.

In "Balancing Hormones with Every Bite," we weave together the threads of nutritional science and emotional well-being. You'll learn about the foods that are not just sustenance but also medicine for your body. Foods rich in fiber, healthy fats, and essential nutrients become the heroes in your quest for hormonal balance.

This subchapter is an invitation to sit at the table with intention, to savor each meal as an act of self-care and love. It's about the quiet moments of reflection when you realize that with every bite, you're taking a step towards a life where PCOS is managed, not feared.

By the end of this subchapter, you'll have more than just a list of hormone-friendly foods; you'll have a deeper understanding of how each meal contributes to your overall well-being. You'll feel empowered, knowing that the choices you make in the kitchen can lead to a more balanced, vibrant life.

Let "Balancing Hormones with Every Bite" be a chapter of hope and healing, a reminder that with every meal, you have the opportunity to nourish not just your body but also your soul.

Chapter 2: Breakfasts to Begin Your Day - A Dawn of Nourishment

As the first light of dawn creeps through your window, a new day beckons—a day full of promise and potential. Chapter 2, "Breakfasts to Begin Your Day," is about embracing the morning with meals that nourish not just your body but also your spirit.

This chapter is an ode to the power of starting your day right, especially when living with PCOS. It's about the quiet moments in the morning when you choose to fuel your body with foods that support your health journey. Each recipe, each ingredient, is chosen with intention, to provide you with the energy and balance needed to face the day with confidence.

"Breakfasts to Begin Your Day" is a collection of recipes that are more than just a means to satiate hunger; they are a ritual of self-care, a daily affirmation of your commitment to your well-being. It's about the emotional satisfaction of preparing a meal that aligns with your body's needs, the joy of flavors that delight your palate, and the peace of mind that comes from knowing you're doing the best for yourself.

We understand that mornings can be a struggle, a time when the symptoms of PCOS can feel overwhelming. This chapter is a gentle reminder that you have the power to set the tone for your day, to choose healing and harmony with every spoonful. It's about the hope that stirs with the steam of your herbal tea, the warmth that spreads with the first bite of your oatmeal, and the strength that builds with each sip of your smoothie.

In "Breakfasts to Begin Your Day," we share stories of resilience and renewal. You'll read about others who have faced the morning with heavy hearts, who have battled fatigue and fought against the tide of PCOS, and who have found solace in the ritual of a nourishing breakfast.

By the end of this chapter, you'll have more than just a collection of breakfast recipes; you'll have a morning routine that empowers you, a series of moments that connect you to your inner strength, and a daily practice that reminds you of the beauty in beginning anew.

Let this chapter be a celebration of new beginnings, a testament to the healing that can happen with the breaking of each day. Embrace the dawn with "Breakfasts to Begin Your Day," and let each morning be a step towards a healthier, happier you.

Energizing Morning Meals - Awakening Your Inner Strength

As the first rays of sunlight gently nudge you awake, a new day unfolds—a blank canvas waiting to be painted with the vibrant colors of life. "Energizing Morning Meals" is the subchapter that invites you to start your day with intention, with meals that awaken your inner strength and kindle the flame of hope within.

This subchapter is a heartfelt tribute to the mornings that can be challenging with PCOS, to the courage it takes to rise each day and face the world with determination. It's about the emotional significance of a morning meal that does more than satisfy hunger—it energizes your spirit and aligns your body with the rhythm of wellness.

We explore the power of breakfast as the first act of self-love each day. It's a quiet declaration that you are worth the time and effort, that your health is a priority. Each recipe is crafted not only to tantalize your taste buds but also to provide the sustained energy needed to thrive despite PCOS.

"Energizing Morning Meals" is an emotional journey through the kitchen, where the sizzle of the pan is a melody of empowerment and the aroma of fresh ingredients is a fragrance of possibility. It's about the joy of crafting a meal that fuels your body's needs, the satisfaction of flavors that dance on your tongue, and the comfort of knowing you're nurturing yourself with every bite.

In this subchapter, we share stories of resilience—of women who have embraced the dawn with weary eyes but hopeful hearts. Their experiences weave into your own, forming a tapestry of shared strength and collective wisdom. You'll find companionship in their tales and inspiration in their triumphs.

As you delve into "Energizing Morning Meals," you'll discover recipes that are more than just food; they are companions on your journey to balance and health. They are reminders that with each new day comes an opportunity for healing and growth.

By the end of this subchapter, you'll have more than just a collection of breakfast ideas; you'll have a morning ritual that fills you with energy and optimism. Let this be the start of your days of empowerment, where each meal is a step towards a life of vitality and joy.
Let "Energizing Morning Meals" be the sunrise in your journey with PCOS, casting light on the path to wellness and illuminating your way to a day filled with energy, hope, and healing.

Quick and Nourishing Smoothies - Blending Comfort and Care

In the rush of the early hours, when time is precious and every moment counts, "Quick and Nourishing Smoothies" offers a reprieve—a chance to pause and nourish yourself with care. This subchapter is a collection of recipes that blend the simplicity of preparation with the complexity of nutrition, all designed to support your journey with PCOS.

Smoothies are more than just a convenient breakfast option; they are a liquid embrace, a soothing blend of ingredients that offer comfort and health in every sip. They are the understanding friend who knows your mornings are hectic, the gentle companion that ensures you don't neglect your well-being amidst the chaos of the dawn.

This subchapter is an emotional ode to the power of a well-crafted smoothie. It's about the reassurance that comes from knowing you can create something both delightful and beneficial in minutes. It's about the vibrant colors of fruits and vegetables that paint your glass with hope, and the rich textures that whisper of self-love and attention.

"Quick and Nourishing Smoothies" is a testament to the small acts of kindness we bestow upon ourselves. It's about the silent victories we celebrate when we choose ingredients that harmonize our hormones and calm our spirits. It's about the joy of discovering that health can be delicious, that taking care of yourself can be as simple as pressing a button on a blender.

In this subchapter, we share the emotional narratives of those who have found solace in the ritual of smoothie-making. Their stories are interwoven with practical advice on how to pack the most nourishing punch into a portable meal. You'll learn about the anti-inflammatory properties of spinach, the hormone-balancing magic of flaxseeds, and the blood-sugar-stabilizing power of berries.

As you explore "Quick and Nourishing Smoothies," you'll feel a connection to each recipe, a sense of camaraderie with every blend. You'll find that these smoothies are not just meals but messages of encouragement, affirmations of your commitment to a life of balance and vitality.

By the end of this subchapter, you'll have a repertoire of recipes that are more than just a means to satiate morning hunger; they are a source of strength and nourishment. Let these smoothies be the quick, comforting start you need, fueling your body and uplifting your spirit as you step into the day.

Let "Quick and Nourishing Smoothies" be your morning ritual of care, a daily reminder that even in the swiftest of moments, you can choose wellness, embrace self-care, and start your day with a heart full of hope and a body brimming with health.

The Serenity of Slow Mornings - Savoring Each Moment

In the gentle embrace of the morning's quiet, when the world still whispers and time seems to stand still, "The Serenity of Slow Mornings" unfolds like a delicate bloom. This subchapter is an invitation to savor each moment, to indulge in the tranquility that a leisurely start can bring to your day, especially when navigating life with PCOS.

Slow mornings are a rare gift, a time to breathe deeply and align your intentions with your actions. They are the soft hours when you can listen to your body's needs and respond with kindness. In this subchapter, we celebrate the luxury of time, the emotional richness of preparing a meal without haste, and the joy of eating with mindfulness and gratitude.

"The Serenity of Slow Mornings" is about the emotional connection we forge with the ritual of breakfast. It's about the steam rising from a cup of herbal tea, carrying with it the scent of hope and the warmth of self-compassion. It's about the sizzle of eggs in a pan, the symphony of a knife chopping fresh vegetables, and the art of plating a meal that is as beautiful to behold as it is healing to consume.

This subchapter is a narrative that honors the struggle against PCOS with every spoonful of yogurt, every slice of avocado, and every sprinkle of chia seeds. It's a testament to the power of starting your day with intention, with foods that balance your hormones and nourish your soul.

In "The Serenity of Slow Mornings," we share stories of those who have found peace in the ritual of a relaxed breakfast. Their journeys become interlaced with yours, offering solace and solidarity. You'll learn that a slow morning is not just a period of time; it's a state of mind, a sacred space where you can find clarity and strength for the day ahead.

As you turn the pages, you'll discover recipes that are crafted to be enjoyed without rush, meals that invite you to linger at the table, to taste each flavor, and to feel each texture. These recipes are more than nourishment; they are a form of self-care, a way to honor your body and your journey with PCOS.

By the end of this subchapter, you'll have more than just a collection of recipes; you'll have a new morning ritual that fills you with serenity and empowerment. Let "The Serenity of Slow Mornings" be a reminder that in the quiet of dawn, there is space for healing, for reflection, and for the gentle unfolding of a day lived with intention and grace.

Let this subchapter guide you to mornings filled with calm, where each bite is a reaffirmation of your commitment to wellness, and each slow breath is a step towards a harmonious life with PCOS.

Chapter 3: Nourishing Lunches for Lasting Energy - The Heartbeat of Your Day

Midday arrives with its bustling energy, a time when the world is fully awake and life moves at a brisk pace. "Nourishing Lunches for Lasting Energy" is the chapter that stands as the heartbeat of your day, offering sustenance to carry you through with vitality and grace, especially when managing PCOS.

This chapter is an emotional embrace, recognizing the midday slump that many with PCOS know all too well—the fatigue that can descend without warning, the hunger that isn't just physical but a deep-seated need for nourishment that satisfies and energizes. It's about the comfort found in a meal that's been prepared with thoughtfulness and care, with ingredients that serve as fuel for both body and soul.

"Nourishing Lunches for Lasting Energy" is a collection of recipes that are more than a mere pause in the day; they are a celebration of life's ongoing dance. Each dish is crafted to provide a steady release of energy, to balance blood sugar levels, and to keep hormones in harmony. It's about the joy of vibrant salads that crunch with life, the warmth of grains that ground you, and the freshness of proteins that build and repair.

This chapter is a narrative of resilience, acknowledging the silent battles fought with every forkful, the determination to choose foods that empower rather than hinder. It's about the emotional journey of living with PCOS, the moments of doubt, and the triumphs of finding a path that leads to wellness.

In "Nourishing Lunches for Lasting Energy," we share the stories of those who have sat down to lunch with heavy hearts but have risen with renewed spirit. Their experiences are woven into the fabric of this chapter, offering solidarity and hope. You'll learn that a nourishing lunch is not just a meal; it's an act of self-care, a midday affirmation of your commitment to health.

As you explore this chapter, you'll find yourself immersed in the art of creating lunches that do more than fill a void; they inspire and rejuvenate. You'll feel a connection to each recipe, a sense of purpose in every choice, and a satisfaction that comes from knowing you're feeding not just your body but also your aspirations for a life free from the constraints of PCOS.

By the end of this chapter, you'll have more than a collection of lunch recipes; you'll have a midday ritual that infuses your day with energy and optimism. Let "Nourishing Lunches for Lasting Energy" be the sustenance for your journey, a daily milestone that marks your progress towards a life of balance, vitality, and joy.

Let this chapter be a reminder that even in the busiest of days, you can find moments of tranquility and nourishment, where each bite is a step towards a healthier, more vibrant you.

Midday Meals to Fuel Your Fire - Igniting Passion with Every Plate

As the clock strikes noon and the sun stands high, it's time to rekindle the embers of your morning energy. "Midday Meals to Fuel Your Fire" is a subchapter dedicated to the meals that reignite your passion and nourish your resolve, especially crucial when you're navigating the complexities of PCOS.

This subchapter is a heartfelt homage to the power of a midday meal to transform your day. It's about the emotional journey from the first bite to the last, the way a carefully crafted lunch can lift your spirits and provide the stamina to continue your fight against PCOS with renewed vigor.

We understand that PCOS can make you feel like you're walking through a fog, where every step is heavy and every breath is a battle. "Midday Meals to Fuel Your Fire" is about clearing that fog with the warmth of wholesome foods, about finding clarity in the nutrients that support your body's delicate balance.

It's an emotional narrative that intertwines the practicality of meal prep with the poetry of eating. It's about the sizzle of lean proteins that promise sustained energy, the crunch of leafy greens that whisper of vitality, and the zest of dressings that speak to the soul. Each recipe is a promise of endurance, a testament to the life-affirming act of nourishing oneself.

In this subchapter, we share stories of those who have sat down to their midday meal with a sense of ritual, who have found in their lunch break a moment of peace amidst the chaos of the day. Their stories are a source of inspiration, a reminder that you're not alone in your journey, and that the simple act of eating can be a profound one.

As you delve into "Midday Meals to Fuel Your Fire," you'll discover that these recipes are more than sustenance; they are a celebration of life's persistent flame. They are an acknowledgment of the inner strength that carries you through the toughest moments, the kind of strength that is nurtured with every mindful mouthful.

By the end of this subchapter, you'll have more than just a collection of lunch recipes; you'll have a midday manifesto, a declaration that with each meal, you're not just eating—you're fueling the fire of your passion for a healthier, more balanced life.

Let "Midday Meals to Fuel Your Fire" be the spark that lights up your day, the warmth that sustains you, and the nourishment that empowers you to face the rest of your day with a heart full of hope and a body brimming with energy.

Salads That Satisfy - A Symphony of Flavors and Feelings

In the heart of the day, when the sun is at its zenith and life buzzes around us, "Salads That Satisfy" offers a moment of respite—a chance to nourish your body and calm your soul with a symphony of flavors and feelings that resonate with the journey of living with PCOS.

This subchapter is a tender narrative about the power of a salad to be more than a dish—it's a canvas of colors, a medley of textures, and a harmony of tastes that together bring satisfaction that goes beyond the palate. It's about the emotional fulfillment that comes from creating a meal that is as pleasing to the eyes as it is healing to the body.

"Salads That Satisfy" is about the quiet triumphs in the choices we make: the crispness of fresh greens that represent vitality, the sweetness of ripe tomatoes that speak of life's simple pleasures, and the crunch of nuts that remind us of the strength we carry within. Each ingredient is selected not just for its nutritional value but for its ability to bring joy and balance to your day.

It's an emotional journey through the textures and tastes of nature's bounty. It's about the comfort found in the ritual of rinsing the vegetables, the mindfulness in slicing them with care, and the artistry in composing a dish that is a feast for the senses. These salads are a celebration of self-care, a testament to the nurturing power of food, and a reflection of the love you pour into your well-being.

In this subchapter, we share stories of connection—of individuals who have found solace in the simplicity of a salad, who have discovered in its layers a metaphor for their own layers of healing and growth. Their stories become a part of your own, a shared experience of finding satisfaction in the wholesome and the natural.

As you explore "Salads That Satisfy," you'll find that these recipes are more than a midday meal; they are a source of comfort and a reminder of the beauty that can be found in the act of nourishing oneself. They are an affirmation of your commitment to a life where PCOS does not overshadow the joy of eating and the pleasure of living.

By the end of this subchapter, you'll have more than just a collection of salad recipes; you'll have a ritual that centers you, a practice that grounds you in the present, and a tradition that fills you with gratitude. Let these salads be the satisfying embrace that carries you through the rest of your day, a reminder that with every forkful, you are taking care of your body and honoring your journey.

Let "Salads That Satisfy" be a chapter of contentment and fulfillment, where each ingredient is a note in the melody of your day, and every salad is a chorus of flavors that sings to your soul.

Warmth in a Bowl: Soups for the Soul - Embracing Comfort and Healing

As the day unfolds and the morning's energy begins to wane, "Warmth in a Bowl: Soups for the Soul" is a subchapter that offers a sanctuary of comfort and healing. It's a collection of recipes that serve as a gentle reminder of the nurturing power of a simple bowl of soup, especially for those navigating the complexities of PCOS.

This subchapter is an emotional homage to the humble soup, a dish that has soothed hearts and warmed bodies through the ages. It's about the solace found in the steam that rises from a hot bowl, the way it carries with it the promise of rest and rejuvenation. Each spoonful is a whisper of care, a testament to the healing that comes from within.

"Warmth in a Bowl" is about the connection we find in the act of cooking—a meditative process where chopping and stirring become a rhythm that grounds us in the present. It's about the anticipation that builds as flavors meld and aromas fill the kitchen, creating a space where worries dissipate and hope simmers.

In this subchapter, we share the emotional narratives of those who have found comfort in the ritual of soup-making. Their stories are interwoven with yours, forming a tapestry of shared experiences. You'll learn that a bowl of soup is not just a meal; it's a companion on chilly days, a healer when the body aches, and a friend when the soul yearns for warmth.

As you delve into "Soups for the Soul," you'll discover recipes that are more than a means to satiate hunger; they are a source of nourishment for both body and spirit. They are an affirmation of your commitment to a life where PCOS is managed with grace and understanding.

By the end of this subchapter, you'll have more than just a collection of soup recipes; you'll have a ritual that fills you with warmth and comfort. Let "Warmth in a Bowl" be the embrace that carries you through the rest of your day, a reminder that with every sip, you are taking care of your body and honoring your journey.

Let this subchapter be a chapter of comfort and healing, where each ingredient is a note in the melody of your day, and every bowl of soup is a chorus of flavors that sings to your soul.

Chapter 4: Dinners to End Your Day on a High Note - A Culinary Crescendo

As the evening sky paints itself with the hues of sunset, it's time to gather around the table for a meal that marks the culmination of your day. "Dinners to End Your Day on a High Note" is a chapter that celebrates the daily symphony of life, especially for those harmonizing the melody of their existence with the rhythm of PCOS.

This chapter is an emotional ode to the dinner table, where the day's stories are shared, and the nourishment of the night begins. It's about the warmth that fills the kitchen as pots simmer and ovens warm, the anticipation of flavors that promise to delight, and the comfort of knowing that each dish supports your journey towards health and balance.

"Dinners to End Your Day on a High Note" is about the joy of cooking as an act of love—for yourself and for those who join you. It's about the satisfaction of creating meals that are not only delicious but also healing, with ingredients that soothe the soul and stabilize the body. Each recipe is a note in the evening's harmony, a blend of nutrients and tastes that sing of wellness and contentment.

It's an emotional journey through the rituals of dinnertime. It's about the clink of cutlery and the clatter of dishes, the laughter and conversations that weave through the steam of a hot meal. These dinners are a celebration of the day's achievements, a time to reflect on the moments of strength and the small victories over PCOS.

In this chapter, we share stories of connection—of families and friends who find solace in the shared experience of a meal, of individuals who draw strength from the solitude of a quiet dinner. Their stories become a part of your own, a shared narrative of nourishment and hope.

As you explore "Dinners to End Your Day on a High Note," you'll discover recipes that are more than a means to end hunger; they are a source of joy and a reminder of the beauty that can be found in the act of eating. They are an affirmation of your commitment to a life where PCOS is a part of the journey, not the destination.

By the end of this chapter, you'll have more than just a collection of dinner recipes; you'll have a nightly tradition that uplifts you, a practice that fills you with gratitude, and a ritual that reminds you of the abundance in your life.

Let "Dinners to End Your Day on a High Note" be the crescendo of your daily symphony, where each ingredient is a note in the melody of your evening, and every meal is a chorus of flavors that sings to your heart.

Comforting Evening Entrees - Nourishing the Heart and Soul

As dusk settles and the evening stars begin their watch, "Comforting Evening Entrees" is a subchapter that speaks to the heart and soul, offering a sanctuary at the end of the day. It's about the meals that wrap you in warmth, the dishes that turn a house into a home, and the recipes that soothe the spirit—especially for those who face the daily challenges of PCOS.

This subchapter is an emotional journey into the kitchen, where the act of cooking becomes a ritual of unwinding and reflection. It's about the comfort found in the familiar sounds of cooking—the gentle bubbling of a stew, the sizzle of a sauté, and the aromatic promise of spices that fill the air with anticipation.

"Comforting Evening Entrees" is about the connection we find in the food we prepare for ourselves and our loved ones. It's about the stories that unfold around the stove, the laughter that echoes against the walls, and the shared glances that say, "We're in this together." Each recipe is a testament to the nurturing power of a well-cooked meal, a reminder that even on the toughest days, there's solace to be found in the simple act of eating.

In this subchapter, we share the emotional narratives of those who have found peace in the ritual of dinnertime. Their stories are interwoven with practical advice on how to create entrees that are not just palatable but also beneficial for managing PCOS. You'll learn that a comforting dinner is not just a meal; it's a moment of respite, a time to nourish your body and acknowledge the efforts of the day.

As you explore "Comforting Evening Entrees," you'll discover recipes that are more than sustenance; they are a source of joy and a reminder of the beauty that can be found in the act of nourishing oneself. They are an affirmation of your commitment to a life where PCOS is a part of the journey, not the destination.

By the end of this subchapter, you'll have more than just a collection of dinner recipes; you'll have a nightly tradition that fills you with warmth and comfort. Let "Comforting Evening Entrees" be the embrace that carries you through the night, a reminder that with every bite, you are taking care of your body and honoring your journey.

Let this subchapter be a chapter of comfort and healing, where each ingredient is a note in the melody of your evening, and every meal is a chorus of flavors that sings to your heart.

Hearty Meals for the Whole Family - Gathering Around the Table

As twilight deepens and the home lights flicker on, "Hearty Meals for the Whole Family" is a subchapter that celebrates the timeless tradition of gathering around the dinner table. It's about the meals that bring us together, the dishes that become the centerpiece of conversation, and the recipes that are passed down through generations—each one carrying the warmth of shared experiences, especially poignant for families touched by PCOS.

This subchapter is an emotional tribute to the family meal, a sacred time when the bustle of the day fades into the background and the focus shifts to the faces and stories that truly matter. It's about the laughter that bubbles up between bites, the supportive glances exchanged over steaming plates, and the collective comfort found in a shared culinary experience.

"Hearty Meals for the Whole Family" is about the connection that food can forge, the way a robust casserole or a tender roast can become a symbol of love and care. Each recipe is crafted with the understanding that those with PCOS need not only nourishment but also the joy and support that come from a family meal. It's about creating dishes that satisfy the body's needs while also catering to the soul's cravings for togetherness and belonging.

In this subchapter, we share the emotional narratives of families who have found strength at the dinner table. Their stories are interwoven with yours, forming a tapestry of shared experiences. You'll learn that a hearty meal is not just about the ingredients; it's about the memories created and the bonds strengthened with every shared meal.

As you explore "Hearty Meals for the Whole Family," you'll discover recipes that are more than sustenance; they are a celebration of life's simple pleasures. They are an affirmation of your commitment to a life where PCOS is a shared journey, not a solitary path.

By the end of this subchapter, you'll have more than just a collection of recipes; you'll have a tradition that enriches your evenings and fortifies your relationships. Let "Hearty Meals for the Whole Family" be the heart of your home, where each dish is a testament to the love and care that fills your space.

Let this subchapter be a chapter of unity and warmth, where each ingredient is a note in the melody of your family's story, and every meal is a chorus of flavors that sings of home, health, and happiness.

Date Night Dishes: PCOS-Friendly Feasts - Savoring Intimacy and Wellness

As the evening whispers sweet nothings and the stars begin their nightly serenade, "Date Night Dishes: PCOS-Friendly Feasts" is a subchapter that intertwines the intimacy of a shared meal with the mindfulness of health. It's about the meals that not only tantalize the taste buds but also honor the body's needs, especially significant for those on a journey with PCOS.

This subchapter is an emotional celebration of connection and care, where the act of preparing a meal becomes an expression of love. It's about the quiet moments in the kitchen, the shared glances and soft smiles as you cook together, and the gentle understanding that every ingredient has been chosen with thoughtfulness and intention.

"Date Night Dishes" is about the joy of creating a feast that is both indulgent and nourishing. It's about finding harmony in flavors that dance together on the plate, creating a symphony that delights the senses and supports well-being. Each recipe is a testament to the balance that can be achieved when wellness and romance are woven together seamlessly.

It's an emotional journey through the courses of a meal shared with someone special. It's about the anticipation that builds with the uncorking of a bottle, the warmth that spreads with the lighting of a candle, and the affection that deepens with each PCOS-friendly bite. These dishes are a celebration of the love that grows stronger when nourished by healthy choices.

In this subchapter, we share the emotional narratives of couples who have found strength and connection in the ritual of a date night dinner. Their stories become a part of your own, a shared narrative of love and health. You'll learn that a date night dish is not just a meal; it's an opportunity for intimacy, a chance to bond over the shared goal of managing PCOS with grace and joy.

As you explore "Date Night Dishes," you'll discover recipes that are more than sustenance; they are a source of connection and a reminder of the beauty that can be found in the act of caring for one another. They are an affirmation of your commitment to a life where PCOS is a shared journey, not a solitary challenge.

By the end of this subchapter, you'll have more than just a collection of recipes; you'll have a tradition that enriches your relationship and nourishes your body. Let "Date Night Dishes: PCOS-Friendly Feasts" be the heart of your evening, where each dish is a testament to the love and care that fills your life.

Let this subchapter be a chapter of intimacy and wellness, where each ingredient is a note in the melody of your love story, and every meal is a chorus of flavors that sings of togetherness and health.

Chapter 5: Snacks and Sides to Keep You Going - The Rhythm of Resilience

As the day marches on, with its myriad tasks and unexpected turns, "Snacks and Sides to Keep You Going" is a chapter that serves as the rhythm of resilience, a culinary beat that keeps you moving in harmony with your body's needs, especially when living with PCOS.

This chapter is an emotional tribute to the small bites and side dishes that are often overlooked yet hold the power to uplift and sustain. It's about the moments of pause, the brief interludes where a handful of nuts or a slice of fruit can become a source of strength, a quiet affirmation of your commitment to health and balance.

"Snacks and Sides to Keep You Going" is about the comfort found in the crunch of a carrot stick, the solace in the smoothness of hummus, and the joy in the juiciness of a ripe berry. Each recipe is a note in the day's melody, a harmonious blend of flavors and nutrients that sing of self-care and attention.

It's an emotional journey through the simple acts of snacking and complementing meals with sides. It's about the mindfulness in choosing foods that nourish without weighing you down, the intention behind selecting ingredients that support your journey with PCOS, and the satisfaction of knowing that each bite is a step towards wellness.

In this chapter, we share the emotional narratives of those who have found solace in the ritual of snacking. Their stories are interwoven with yours, forming a tapestry of shared experiences. You'll learn that a snack or a side dish is not just a quick bite; it's a moment of nourishment, a chance to refuel and recharge.

As you explore "Snacks and Sides to Keep You Going," you'll discover recipes that are more than a mere accompaniment to meals; they are a celebration of life's ongoing journey. They are an affirmation of your commitment to a life where PCOS is a part of the path, not an obstacle.

By the end of this chapter, you'll have more than just a collection of recipes; you'll have a rhythm that carries you through the day, a practice that fills you with energy, and a tradition that reminds you of the joy in the little things.

Let "Snacks and Sides to Keep You Going" be the melody that plays in the background of your day, where each ingredient is a note in the harmony of your life, and every snack is a chorus of flavors that sings of vitality and joy.

Guilt-Free Grazing - Savoring Mindfulness in Every Morsel

In the ebb and flow of daily life, "Guilt-Free Grazing" is a subchapter that celebrates the art of snacking without remorse, especially for those on the journey of managing PCOS. It's about the small, mindful choices that nourish not just the body but also the soul.

This subchapter is an emotional exploration of the moments between meals, the times when hunger whispers and the heart seeks a gentle reprieve. It's about the joy found in a crisp apple, the solace in a handful of almonds, and the comfort in the smoothness of a perfectly ripe avocado. Each snack is a choice made with intention, a deliberate act of kindness towards oneself.

"Guilt-Free Grazing" is about transforming the act of snacking from a mindless habit into a mindful ritual. It's about the connection with the food you eat, the appreciation of its origin, and the gratitude for the nourishment it provides. It's about the peace that comes from knowing you're grazing on foods that align with your body's needs, supporting your PCOS management with every bite.

In this subchapter, we share the emotional stories of those who have found balance in their snacking habits. Their experiences are interwoven with practical advice on how to choose snacks that satisfy without guilt. You'll learn that guilt-free grazing is not just about eating; it's about savoring the flavors, textures, and the very act of nourishment.

As you delve into "Guilt-Free Grazing," you'll discover recipes and ideas that are more than quick fixes for hunger; they are a source of joy and a reminder of the beauty that can be found in the act of eating mindfully. They are an affirmation of your commitment to a life where PCOS is a part of the journey, not a barrier to enjoyment.

By the end of this subchapter, you'll have more than just a collection of snack ideas; you'll have a new perspective on grazing, a practice that fills you with contentment, and a tradition that reminds you of the importance of self-care.

Let "Guilt-Free Grazing" be the melody that plays softly in the background of your day, where each snack is a note in the harmony of your health, and every mindful choice sings of vitality and self-compassion.

Sides That Steal the Show - The Unsung Heroes of the Table

As the day's narrative unfolds, with its peaks and valleys, "Sides That Steal the Show" is a subchapter that honors the unsung heroes of the table—the side dishes that, while often playing a supporting role, possess the power to elevate a meal from ordinary to extraordinary, especially for those balancing the nuances of PCOS.

This subchapter is an emotional tribute to the side dishes that do more than just accompany a main course; they tell their own story, they add depth and dimension to every meal, and they resonate with the care and attention poured into their creation. It's about the vibrancy of roasted vegetables that add color to the plate, the rustic charm of a perfectly baked sweet potato, and the elegance of a quinoa salad dressed in a light vinaigrette.

"Sides That Steal the Show" is about the connection we find in the shared experience of a meal, where every component on the plate plays a part in the symphony of flavors. It's about the pride in preparing a dish that might not take center stage but still receives the applause, the satisfaction of knowing that these sides are crafted with ingredients that support your health and well-being.

In this subchapter, we share the emotional narratives of those who have found joy in the simplicity of a side dish. Their stories are interwoven with yours, forming a tapestry of shared experiences. You'll learn that a side dish is not just an addition to a meal; it's a moment of nourishment, an opportunity to indulge in the diversity of textures and tastes that nature offers.

As you explore "Sides That Steal the Show," you'll discover recipes that are more than accompaniments; they are a celebration of the bounty of the earth. They are an affirmation of your commitment to a life where PCOS is managed with grace and where every meal is an opportunity to nourish and delight.

By the end of this subchapter, you'll have more than just a collection of side dish recipes; you'll have a new appreciation for the elements that round out a meal, a practice that fills you with gratitude, and a tradition that reminds you of the richness of culinary diversity.

Let "Sides That Steal the Show" be the melody that harmonizes with the main course, where each side dish is a note in the harmony of your dining experience, and every recipe is a chorus of flavors that sings of creativity, health, and joy.

Sweet Treats Without the Spike - Indulging in Wholesome Decadence

As the day winds down and we seek solace in the sweetness of life, "Sweet Treats Without the Spike" is a subchapter that offers a guiltless indulgence, a way to savor the richness of desserts without the worry of disrupting the delicate balance of PCOS.

This subchapter is an emotional journey into the world of desserts that are not only delectable but also mindful of your health. It's about the moments of pure joy when you bite into a fluffy muffin or a slice of creamy cheesecake, knowing that these treats are crafted to nourish as much as they are to delight. It's about the satisfaction of a sweet craving met without the aftermath of a sugar spike.

"Sweet Treats Without the Spike" is about the connection we find in the act of treating ourselves. It's about the love poured into every mix and stir, the anticipation of a dessert that's both scrumptious and supportive of your PCOS management. Each recipe is a testament to the possibility of having it all—the sweetness of life without the compromise on health.

In this subchapter, we share the emotional narratives of those who have found a way to indulge without guilt. Their stories are interwoven with yours, forming a tapestry of shared experiences. You'll learn that a sweet treat is not just a dessert; it's a celebration of balance, a moment of self-care, and a testament to the creativity that thrives within the constraints of dietary mindfulness.

As you explore "Sweet Treats Without the Spike," you'll discover recipes that are more than a conclusion to a meal; they are a source of happiness and a reminder of the beauty that can be found in the act of indulgence. They are an affirmation of your commitment to a life where PCOS is a part of the journey, not a deterrent to enjoyment.

By the end of this subchapter, you'll have more than just a collection of dessert recipes; you'll have a new perspective on sweets, a practice that fills you with delight, and a tradition that reminds you of the importance of treating yourself with kindness and joy.

Let "Sweet Treats Without the Spike" be the melody that plays softly in the background of your day, where each dessert is a note in the harmony of your health, and every mindful indulgence sings of vitality and self-compassion.

Chapter 6: Healing from the Inside Out - Embracing Wholeness and Harmony

As the twilight of your journey with PCOS beckons, "Healing from the Inside Out" is a chapter that speaks to the deepest part of your being. It's about the holistic approach to wellness, where healing is not just a physical process but an emotional and spiritual one as well.

This chapter is an emotional testament to the power of inner transformation. It's about the realization that true healing begins within, that every choice you make—from the food you eat to the thoughts you nurture—has the potential to bring you closer to the harmony you seek. It's about the courage to look beyond the symptoms and the treatments, to the core of your health and happiness.

"Healing from the Inside Out" is about the connection between mind, body, and spirit. It's about the quiet moments of introspection, the gentle acceptance of your body's signals, and the compassionate understanding of your own needs. Each section of this chapter is a step on the path to self-discovery, a journey towards a balanced and fulfilled life.

It's an emotional journey through the layers of self-care. It's about the warmth of a cup of herbal tea that calms the mind, the grounding effect of a walk in nature, and the restorative power of a good night's sleep. These practices are the unsung melodies of healing, the subtle rhythms that, when combined, create a symphony of well-being.

In this chapter, we share the emotional narratives of those who have embraced their journey with PCOS with open hearts. Their stories are interwoven with practical advice on how to cultivate a lifestyle that supports holistic healing. You'll learn that healing from the inside out is not just about managing a condition; it's about nurturing a life that is rich, vibrant, and deeply connected to the essence of who you are.

As you explore "Healing from the Inside Out," you'll discover that this chapter is more than a conclusion to a book; it's the beginning of a new chapter in your life. It's an affirmation of your commitment to a journey of health that is comprehensive, compassionate, and conscious.

By the end of this chapter, you'll have more than just a collection of holistic practices; you'll have a new perspective on health, a practice that fills you with peace, and a tradition that reminds you of the interconnectedness of all aspects of your being.

Let "Healing from the Inside Out" be the gentle whisper that guides you to wholeness, where each practice is a note in the harmony of your existence, and every step is a dance of joy and self-compassion.

Foods as Medicine - The Healing Harmony of Nature

In the quiet corners of our lives, where the whispers of well-being are often lost in the noise of the day, "Foods as Medicine" is a subchapter that brings us back to the roots of healing. It's a heartfelt exploration of the ancient wisdom that sees food not just as sustenance, but as a key to unlocking the body's natural ability to heal, especially poignant for those on the journey with PCOS.

This subchapter is an emotional ode to the foods that have the power to act as medicine. It's about the deep respect for the nutrients that nature provides, the understanding that within every fruit, vegetable, seed, and nut lies a potential remedy for the ailments that challenge us. It's about the connection we forge with each meal, knowing that what we eat can become a part of our healing process.

"Foods as Medicine" is about the silent dialogue between our bodies and the foods we choose. It's about the moments of realization when we recognize the impact of a balanced diet on our hormonal health, the gentle acknowledgment of the anti-inflammatory properties of a spice, or the blood sugar-stabilizing effects of a fiber-rich grain. Each ingredient is chosen with intention, a deliberate step towards harmony and health.

In this subchapter, we share the emotional narratives of those who have turned to their kitchens for healing. Their stories are interwoven with practical advice on how to incorporate medicinal foods into daily life. You'll learn that food as medicine is not just a concept; it's a practice, a way of life, and a path to empowerment.

As you delve into "Foods as Medicine," you'll discover recipes and insights that are more than just dietary guidelines; they are a source of hope and a reminder of the power that lies in the choices we make. They are an affirmation of your commitment to a life where PCOS is managed with wisdom, care, and the healing harmony of nature.

By the end of this subchapter, you'll have more than just a collection of nutritional facts; you'll have a new perspective on eating, a practice that fills you with peace, and a tradition that reminds you of the profound connection between food and wellness.

Let "Foods as Medicine" be the melody that resonates with the rhythm of your body, where each food is a note in the harmony of your health, and every meal is a chorus of flavors that sings of restoration and balance.

Lifestyle Changes for Lasting Impact - Crafting a Symphony of Self-Care

In the quiet afterglow of personal reflection, "Lifestyle Changes for Lasting Impact" is a subchapter that resonates with the profound truth that healing is a holistic symphony, where every aspect of our lives plays a crucial part in the melody of our well-being, especially when harmonizing with PCOS.

This subchapter is an emotional narrative about the transformative power of lifestyle changes. It's about the courage to embrace new habits, the strength to let go of those that no longer serve us, and the wisdom to craft a daily rhythm that supports our deepest health needs. It's about the realization that every choice—from the moment we wake to the moment we rest—composes the unique symphony of our lives.

"Lifestyle Changes for Lasting Impact" is about the connection we forge with our routines, the peace that comes from aligning our actions with our values, and the joy of discovering a lifestyle that fosters balance and vitality. Each section of this chapter is a note in the harmony of self-care, a step towards a life where PCOS is not a dissonant chord but a part of the music that makes us who we are.

It's an emotional journey through the layers of change. It's about the warmth of the morning sun on our skin as we exercise, the grounding effect of mindful breathing, and the restorative power of connecting with loved ones. These practices are the unsung melodies of healing, the subtle rhythms that, when combined, create a symphony of well-being.

In this chapter, we share the emotional narratives of those who have embraced their journey with PCOS with open hearts. Their stories are interwoven with practical advice on how to cultivate a lifestyle that supports holistic healing. You'll learn that lifestyle changes for lasting impact are not just about managing a condition; they're about nurturing a life that is rich, vibrant, and deeply connected to the essence of who you are.

As you explore "Lifestyle Changes for Lasting Impact," you'll discover that this chapter is more than a conclusion to a book; it's the beginning of a new chapter in your life. It's an affirmation of your commitment to a journey of health that is comprehensive, compassionate, and conscious.

By the end of this chapter, you'll have more than just a collection of holistic practices; you'll have a new perspective on health, a practice that fills you with peace, and a tradition that reminds you of the interconnectedness of all aspects of your being.

Let "Lifestyle Changes for Lasting Impact" be the gentle whisper that guides you to wholeness, where each practice is a note in the harmony of your existence, and every step is a dance of joy and self-compassion.

Beyond the Kitchen: A Holistic Approach to PCOS - Embracing the Full Spectrum of Self-Care

As the day's light fades into the soft glow of evening, "Beyond the Kitchen: A Holistic Approach to PCOS" is a subchapter that extends a hand beyond the boundaries of dietary guidance, reaching into the vast expanse of holistic self-care. It's about the understanding that managing PCOS is a journey that encompasses more than what we eat—it's about how we live, think, and care for our entire being.

This subchapter is an emotional acknowledgment of the intricate tapestry of life with PCOS. It's about the realization that every aspect of our lives—our stress levels, sleep patterns, relationships, and even our thoughts—can have a profound impact on our health. It's about the courage to embrace change, not just in the kitchen but in all corners of our existence.

"Beyond the Kitchen" is about the connection we find in the quiet moments of self-reflection, the peace that comes from a mindful meditation session, and the joy of connecting with others who understand our journey. Each practice introduced in this chapter is a note in the harmony of holistic care, a step towards a life where PCOS is managed with grace and wisdom.

It's an emotional journey through the layers of self-care. It's about the warmth of a yoga mat beneath your feet, the grounding effect of deep breathing, and the restorative power of laughter and love. These practices are the unsung melodies of healing, the subtle rhythms that, when combined, create a symphony of well-being.

In this chapter, we share the emotional narratives of those who have embraced their journey with PCOS with open hearts. Their stories are interwoven with practical advice on how to cultivate a lifestyle that supports holistic healing. You'll learn that a holistic approach to PCOS is not just about managing a condition; it's about nurturing a life that is rich, vibrant, and deeply connected to the essence of who you are.

As you explore "Beyond the Kitchen," you'll discover that this chapter is more than a conclusion to a book; it's the beginning of a new chapter in your life. It's an affirmation of your commitment to a journey of health that is comprehensive, compassionate, and conscious.

By the end of this chapter, you'll have more than just a collection of holistic practices; you'll have a new perspective on health, a practice that fills you with peace, and a tradition that reminds you of the interconnectedness of all aspects of your being.

Let "Beyond the Kitchen: A Holistic Approach to PCOS" be the gentle whisper that guides you to wholeness, where each practice is a note in the harmony of your existence, and every step is a dance of joy and self-compassion.

Conclusion: The Path Forward - Living and Thriving with PCOS

As we reach the final pages of this journey, the "Conclusion" is not an end but a beginning—a threshold to a life lived with awareness, care, and a deepened understanding of PCOS. It's a chapter that weaves together the threads of knowledge, emotion, and experience into a tapestry of hope and empowerment.

This conclusion is an emotional embrace, acknowledging the challenges you've faced and the strength you've garnered along the way. It's about the realization that living with PCOS is not just about managing symptoms but about thriving in spite of them. It's about the courage to continue on a path that is sometimes rocky, the resilience to rise with each dawn, and the joy of knowing that you are not alone.

"The Path Forward" is about the connection we find in our shared stories, the comfort in knowing that others walk beside us, and the inspiration we draw from each other's victories. It's about the collective wisdom that comes from a community of souls who understand the nuances of this condition.

It's an emotional journey that extends beyond the kitchen, beyond the pages of this book, and into the very fabric of your daily life. It's about the small acts of self-care that become grand gestures of self-love, the mindful choices that become second nature, and the habits that form the foundation of a life lived in harmony with PCOS.

In this conclusion, we share the emotional narratives of those who have embraced their journey with open hearts. Their stories are interwoven with the practical advice and the holistic practices you've explored throughout the book. You'll learn that the conclusion is not just a summary; it's a promise, a promise to yourself that the journey continues, that every day is an opportunity for growth and healing.

As you reflect on "The Path Forward," you'll discover that this conclusion is more than a final chapter; it's a new perspective on life, a practice that fills you with hope, and a tradition that reminds you of the power you hold within.

Let "The Path Forward" be the gentle nudge that guides you to embrace your PCOS journey fully, where each step is a note in the harmony of your existence, and every breath is a dance of joy and self-compassion. Here's to living and thriving with PCOS, to the days ahead filled with health, happiness, and the sweet melody of a life well-lived.

Your PCOS Journey: A Tapestry of Triumphs

Your journey with PCOS is a tapestry woven with threads of courage, resilience, and hope. It's a story that unfolds with each day, each challenge faced, and each triumph earned. This tapestry is rich with the colors of your experiences, the patterns of your struggles, and the textures of your victories.

"Your PCOS Journey: A Tapestry of Triumphs" is an emotional reflection on the path you've walked since the moment of diagnosis. It's about the tears shed in frustration, the smiles that broke through on good days, and the laughter that echoed on the days when you felt triumphant. It's about the strength you found in yourself when you thought there was none left, the determination that grew with every setback, and the wisdom that came from each lesson learned.

This tapestry is not just a personal keepsake; it's a beacon for others who walk a similar path. It's a testament to the fact that while PCOS may be a part of your life, it does not define you. Each thread represents a choice, a change, a moment of understanding—a holistic approach that encompasses not just the physical aspects of PCOS, but the emotional and spiritual as well.

In "Your PCOS Journey," we share the emotional narratives of those who have woven their own tapestries. Their stories are interwoven with yours, creating a quilt of shared experiences. You'll learn that this journey is not just about managing a condition; it's about embracing a life that is textured, vibrant, and deeply connected to the essence of who you are.

As you reflect on your tapestry of triumphs, you'll see more than a collection of experiences; you'll see a masterpiece that tells a story of endurance, growth, and self-love. It's a reminder that every challenge faced is a triumph in its own right, and every day lived with intention is a stroke of beauty on the canvas of life.

Let "Your PCOS Journey: A Tapestry of Triumphs" be the narrative that inspires you to continue weaving your story, where each thread is a note in the harmony of your existence, and every triumph is a testament to your spirit and your will to thrive. Here's to the tapestry you're creating—one that is as unique and beautiful as you are.